Arterial Blood Gas Analysis
An easy learning guide

Arterial Blood Gas Analysis

An easy learning guide

Fiona Foxall MA, RGN, ENB100, DPSN, BSc, PGCE

Head of Division, Continuing Development,
School of Health, University of Wolverhampton,
West Midlands, UK

With original artwork by Helen Blackburn

Arterial Blood Gas Analysis: An Easy Learning Guide
Fiona Foxall

ISBN: 978-1-905539-04-8

First published 2008,
Reprinted in 2011

British Library Catalogue in Publication Data
A catalogue record for this book is available from the British Library

Notice
Clinical practice and medical knowledge constantly evolve. Standard safety precautions
must be followed, but, as knowledge is broadened by research, changes in practice,
treatment and drug therapy may become necessary or appropriate. Readers must check
the most current product information provided by the manufacturer of each drug to be
administered and verify the dosages and correct administration, as well as contraindications.
It is the responsibility of the practitioner, utilising the experience and knowledge of the
patient, to determine dosages and the best treatment for each individual patient. Any
brands mentioned in this book are as examples only and are not endorsed by the Publisher.
Neither the Publisher nor the author assume any liability for any injury and/or damage to
persons or property arising from this publication.

The Publisher
To contact M&K Publishing write to:
M&K Update Ltd · The Old Bakery · St. John's Street
Keswick · Cumbria CA12 5AS
Tel: 01768 773030 · Fax: 01768 781099
publishing@mkupdate.co.uk
www.mkupdate.co.uk

Copyedited, indexed, designed and typeset in AdGaramond 10/12 by S. Maria Hampshire.
Cover design and graphics by Luke Kelsey.

Printed in England by Ferguson Print (Keswick) Ltd.

DEDICATION

This work is dedicated to the late D. Kendal Williams:

You gave me wings.
Thank you.

Contents

Acknowledgements

I would like to thank my special friends and family for their help with this workbook, especially:

Ann Donnellan and Megan Tanner for their initial and ongoing feedback on this work, which altered my views – and the work – considerably; Professor Rebecca Jester for her gentle but forceful push to make me do it; Kate Deacon for the time she took to read the draft and for her helpful comments; Helen Blackburn for her fabulous artistry which was put to good use for the illustrations; and Chris Blackburn and Matthew Blackburn for helping me to format the material.

What would I have done without you all.

Introduction

Blood gas analysis is one of the most frequently requested blood tests when caring for the critically ill patient, as it provides very valuable information about the respiratory and acid–base status of the patient (Shoulders-Odom, 2000).

However, many healthcare professionals find it difficult to get to grips with blood gas analysis. It often seems complex and daunting, but if you work your way through this book and carry out all the exercises, you will soon become confident and competent at analysing blood gases and will understand all the information that initially seemed so complicated.

Blood gas analysis is a skill which requires continuous practice, so once you have completed this workbook keep analysing blood gases as often as you can and discuss your findings with your mentor, until it becomes easy. I promise you, with practice it will.

Here's to easy learning!

How to use this workbook

Start at the beginning. Even if you are feeling quite happy about blood gas analysis, it will be good revision for you. Work steadily through all the material, ensuring you understand the information in each chapter before moving on to the next.

Once you have read each chapter complete the *Consolidation* section at the end. This will help you understand the information sufficiently. As you work through Chapter 4 you should answer the questions as you go. It will be helpful if you can find a mentor to help with any exercises you are unsure about.

If you don't know a particular answer, do try to work it out by remembering the information you have already read. If you still can't work it out, try discussing it with your chosen mentor. If it is still not clear, then look up the answer in the *Answer and Teaching Notes* section at the back of the workbook. This section should be used as a last resort, for checking purposes only. You will learn far more by working things out for yourself, rather than by looking at the answers that have been provided. If you do have to look up an answer, make sure you understand it – don't just accept it. Remember to discuss any problems with your mentor.

If you already have a reasonable knowledge and understanding of blood gas analysis, you could – if you wish – attempt the *Consolidation* sections *before* reading the explanatory text. This will give you a very good idea of your current level of knowledge and will also identify any gaps in your knowledge, which you can then concentrate on filling.

Aims of this workbook

This book aims to extend your knowledge and clinical application of arterial blood gas analysis.

After completing this workbook you will be able to:

- State the normal values of blood gases.
- Define each parameter and understand its significance.
- Discuss gas transport in the blood.
- Briefly discuss acid–base balance.
- Identify the steps for safely obtaining an arterial sample of blood.
- Determine if there is acidosis or alkalosis present.
- Determine whether disturbances are respiratory or metabolic.
- Discuss the term 'compensation' in relation to blood gas analysis.
- State the possible causes of abnormal blood gases.
- Discuss what actions are appropriate for different abnormalities.

Chapter 1

The parameters

The majority of critically ill patients need to have analysis of their blood gases and you need to be able to interpret the results. Firstly, we will consider which parameters are examined, describe their normal values, and explain what they mean.

Acidity and alkalinity (pH)

Hydrogen is an end-product of cellular metabolism. pH is directly proportional to the hydrogen (H) ion concentration and measures the acidity or alkalinity of a substance (Haworth *et al.*, 2004). The pH scale is a continuum from a value of 1 to 14, with 7 in the middle (see Fig. 1.1).

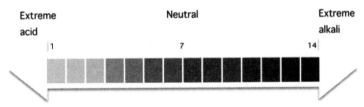

Extreme acid	Neutral	Extreme alkali
1	7	14

Fig. 1.1 *The pH scale.*

A pH of 1 is strongly acidic, a pH of 14 is strongly alkaline, and a pH of 7 is neutral. Water is a neutral substance. Blood has a pH of 7.35–7.45, so it is very slightly alkaline. However, even when the pH of blood is 7.0 (neutral on the pH scale) it is very 'acidic', because a pH of 7.0 indicates an increase of hydrogen ions well above the upper limit of normal (45 nmol/L) (see Chapter 3). Patients with this pH would be extremely acidotic and in need of urgent treatment.

The term pH is a mathematical expression relating to the amount of free hydrogen ions present and it is a negative logarithm:

$$pH\,6 = 1 \times 10^{-6} = 0.000001$$
$$pH\,7 = 1 \times 10^{-7} = 0.0000001$$

It is not important to remember these equations, but what is important is knowing that a change in pH from pH 7 to pH 6 represents a *tenfold* change in the actual number of hydrogen ions present (Bruck *et al.*, 2005) – or put more simply, hydrogen ions affect the pH of the blood, and a relatively small change in pH is dangerous for the patient.

Partial pressure (P)

The letter 'P' in PO_2 and PCO_2 stands for partial pressure. You may have seen these parameters expressed as PaO_2 and PAO_2 and $PaCO_2$ and $PACO_2$. The small 'a' stands for *arterial* and the capital 'A' stands for *alveolar*. Generally, PaO_2 and $PaCO_2$ are expressed with the small 'a' as we examine *arterial* blood gases. However, in practice the 'a' is not usually used very much and you will see the terms PO_2 and PCO_2 far more often. Dalton's Law explains the term 'partial pressure'.

Dalton's Law

Each gas in a mixture exerts a partial pressure that is relative to its concentration in the mixture (Viney, 1999). Adding together all partial pressures exerted by each gas gives the total pressure of the mixture.

Air is made up of nitrogen (N_2), oxygen (O_2), carbon dioxide (CO_2) and water (H_2O) vapour:

$$O_2 + CO_2 + N_2 + H_2O = Air$$

All of these exert a partial pressure. If the pressure of the oxygen is added to the pressure of the nitrogen, carbon dioxide and water vapour, the sum total is 760 mmHg, which is **atmospheric pressure**.

Table 1.1 Partial pressures of oxygen, carbon dioxide, nitrogen and water in air

	Oxygen (O_2)	Carbon dioxide (CO_2)	Nitrogen (N_2)	Water vapour (H_2O)	Total in air
%	20.84	0.04	78.62	0.5	100
mmHg	158.4	0.3	597.5	3.8	760
kPa	21.12	0.04	79.6	0.5	101.26

Therefore PO_2 and PCO_2 are the measurements of the partial pressures which oxygen and carbon dioxide exert in the blood. PO_2 and PCO_2 are measured either in kiloPascals (kPa) or in millimetres of mercury (mmHg). You will find both measurements throughout this workbook.

> **Converting between kPa and mmHg**
> To change kPa to mmHg – multiply by 7.5
> To change mmHg to kPa – divide by 7.5
> *(Jevon and Ewens, 2002)*

Example:

To convert a PO_2 of 10.83 kPa into mmHg
Multiply 10.83 by 7.5
$10.83 \times 7.5 = 81.225$ mmHg

Partial pressure of oxygen (PO$_2$)

PO$_2$ is the measurement of the partial pressure of oxygen that is dissolved in the plasma of the blood, which is usually less than 3% of the total oxygen in the blood (the rest being carried by haemoglobin, the pigment found in red blood cells) (Janson-Cohen, 2005). We will consider this in more detail later.

The PO$_2$ gives no indication of the acid–base status of the body, but clearly gives an indication of oxygen uptake and therefore the respiratory status of the patient as it demonstrates the efficiency of gaseous exchange.

> **Normal PO$_2$**
> 10.6–13.3 kPa *or* 80–100 mmHg

Partial pressure of carbon dioxide (PCO$_2$)

PCO$_2$ is the measurement of the partial pressure of carbon dioxide that is dissolved in the blood. When carbon dioxide is dissolved in water (as it is, as a result of metabolism) it changes into carbonic acid which, if not dealt with by the body, causes a respiratory acidosis. Therefore, the higher the PCO$_2$, the more acidotic the patient becomes. In terms of blood gas analysis, the PCO$_2$ is referred to as the respiratory component as it is indicative of ventilation.

> **Normal PCO$_2$**
> 4.6–6.0 kPa *or* 35–45 mmHg

Bicarbonate (HCO₃)

We need to know the amount of bicarbonate in the blood because 70% of CO_2 is carried in this form from the tissues to the lungs for excretion. It is calculated by the blood gas analyser from measurement of pH and PCO_2.

Some blood gas analysers measure both the actual and standard bicarbonate. The standard bicarbonate is the calculated bicarbonate taking the PCO_2 at a standard 5.6 kPa and is the more important parameter of the two.

Bicarbonate is referred to as the metabolic component.

> **Normal HCO₃**
> 22–26 mmol/L

Base excess (BE)

Rising levels of bicarbonate make the blood more alkaline and a depletion of bicarbonate renders the blood more acidic. Base excess refers to the amount of base (alkali) which needs to be added to, or taken away from, the blood to return the pH to 7.4 (Mattson-Porth, 2005).

We cannot take bicarbonate away from the blood but it is easy to add, although this is rarely done as it may precipitate cellular acidosis and a left shift of the oxygen dissociation curve (see Chapter 2) resulting in decreased oxygen delivery (Resuscitation Council UK, 2000).

Base excess is not a tangible substance (as are the other measured parameters) but it represents how much the body is using the buffering systems to maintain normal pH (see Chapter 3).

Base excess is also calculated by the blood gas analyser.

• *If the bicarbonate is high*, the amount of base (alkali) in the blood will be excessive and therefore the base reading will be strongly positive, that is, a base excess (Mattson-Porth, 2005).

• *If the bicarbonate is low,* there is a base deficit and the reading will be negative (Mattson-Porth, 2005).

Therefore the value of base excess should ideally be 0 as there should be neither an excess nor a deficit of base. However, this is rarely the case.

Normal base excess (BE)

−2 to +2

Oxygen saturation (SaO₂)

This refers to the amount of oxygen being carried by the haemoglobin (Hb) molecules. The haemoglobin molecule is divided into two portions: a globin portion (made up of protein) and a haem portion (made up of iron). The haem portion is further divided into four areas on the molecule (see Fig. 1.2).

Each haem portion is capable of carrying one oxygen molecule. If all haem portions are carrying one oxygen molecule, the haemoglobin is 100% saturated. This usually only occurs when breathing oxygen-enriched air. The normal oxygen saturation is 97% because 97% of oxygen is carried by the haemoglobin (the other 3% is carried in the plasma in a dissolved form).

• Each gram of haemoglobin (if 100% saturated) carries 1.34 mL of oxygen.
• Each red blood cell contains around 250 million haemoglobin molecules and is capable of carrying more than a billion oxygen molecules (Janson-Cohen, 2005).

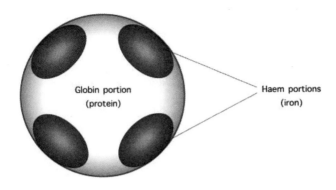

Fig. 1.2 *The haemoglobin molecule.*

- There are over 5 million red blood cells in every mL of blood.
- Each 100 mL of arterial blood can carry 20 mL of oxygen.

The actual amount of oxygen carried by the blood depends on the amount of haemoglobin present, but just because a patient is 100% saturated does not necessarily mean that enough oxygen is available to the tissues. If haemoglobin is low, there will be less oxygen carrying capacity – even if oxygen saturation levels are high. So, patients can be hypoxic when oxygen saturation levels are normal.

Consider two patients, both of whom have an oxygen saturation of 92%, but patient 1 has a haemoglobin of 14 g/dL (grams per decilitre) and patient 2 has a haemoglobin of 7 g/dL. Patient 1 will be carrying more oxygen in the blood, simply because there is more haemoglobin present, and therefore has the higher oxygen-carrying capacity.

Consolidation

See pages 71–72 for answers

1.1 Write down the blood gas parameters that are measured and their normal values, including the units in which they are measured:

_____

_____

_____

1.2 What does pH measure?

_____

1.3 Is a pH of 3 acidic or alkaline?

_____

1.4 Is a pH of 11 acidic or alkaline?

_____

1.5 Name a pH-neutral substance:

_____

1.6 Is blood normally slightly acidic or slightly alkaline?

_____

1.7 Which end-product of cellular metabolism affects blood pH?

_____

1.8 What does the 'a' in PaO_2 stand for?

_____

1.9 What does the 'A' in $PACO_2$ stand for?

_____

1.10 What does 'P' in PO_2 and PCO_2 stand for?

_____

1.11 Explain the term partial pressure:

_____

_____

_____

1.12 Convert 9.98 kPa to mmHg:

_____

1.13 Convert 45.3 mmHg to kPa:

_____

1.14 Does the level of oxygen in blood affect the acid–base status of the patient?

_____

1.15 When CO_2 is dissolved in water, what is the name of the compound formed?

_____

1.16 What percentage of CO_2 is carried to the lungs by HCO_3?

_____

1.17 If there is a base excess, will the level of HCO_3 be high or low?

_____

1.18 If there is a base deficit, will the level of HCO_3 be high or low?

_____

1.19 Does oxygen saturation measure the oxygen that is dissolved in the plasma or the oxygen that is being carried by the haemoglobin?

_____

1.20 Which substance makes up the 'haem' portion of the haemoglobin molecule?

_____

1.21 Which substance makes up the 'globin' portion of the haemoglobin molecule?

_____

1.22 How many oxygen molecules can one haemoglobin molecule carry?

_____

1.23 If one haemoglobin molecule is carrying three oxygen molecules, what will be the percentage oxygen saturation?

_____

1.24 How many mL of oxygen is 1 g of haemoglobin carrying if it is 100% saturated?

_____

1.25 Patient 1 has an Hb of 11.6 g/dL and SaO_2 of 98%. Patient 2 has an Hb of 13.2 g/dL and SaO_2 of 96%. Which patient has the greater oxygen carrying capacity?

_____

Notes

Chapter 2

Gas transport

Before considering specific disturbances in acid–base balance, we should first explore how gases are normally transported in the blood.

Oxygen transport

Oxygen is transported in two ways:

- in the form of oxyhaemoglobin
- in dissolved form.

Around 97% of oxygen is transported in the form of oxyhaemoglobin, where the oxygen molecule is attached to haemoglobin.

Less than 3% is transported in the plasma in a dissolved form. It might seem a very small amount but it is very important because dissolved oxygen exerts the partial pressure.

A low oxygen saturation indicates a *VQ mismatch*.

VQ mismatch

This means there is a mismatch of ventilation and perfusion in the lungs, so that blood goes to parts of the lungs that are not oxygenated and/or there is a lack of perfusion to the parts of the lungs where oxygen is available. Therefore, deoxygenated blood is shunted through the lungs without being able to pick up oxygen.

Oxygen dissociation

It is useful to be able to measure the partial pressure of oxygen (PO_2) as there is a direct relationship between this and oxygen saturation, as illustrated in the oxygen dissociation curve (see Fig. 2.1). The curve highlights the affinity of oxygen for haemoglobin.

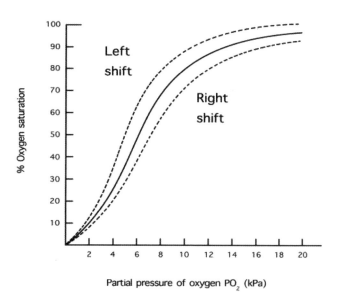

Partial pressure of oxygen PO_2 (kPa)

Fig. 2.1 *Oxygen dissociation curve showing shifts to the left and right of the normal curve.*

High PO_2

When PO_2 is high, oxygen is strongly affiliated to haemoglobin, so oxygen saturation will also be high. That simply means that when blood arrives at the lungs and oxygen affinity for haemoglobin is high, the blood will pick up a lot of oxygen – hence PO_2 and O_2 saturation are high. There is a problem here, however, because when the blood arrives at the tissues, oxygen affinity for haemoglobin remains high, so it is more difficult for the oxygen to be released into the tissues. This happens when there is a shift to the left of the curve, which occurs during alkalosis. This explains why alkalotic patients can have a good PO_2 and O_2 saturation yet may look pallid or even cyanosed.

Low PO_2

When PO_2 is low, there is less affinity of oxygen for haemoglobin, so oxygen saturation drops. Thus, when blood arrives at the lungs and oxygen affinity to haemoglobin is low, the blood will pick up less oxygen – hence PO_2 and O_2 saturation are low. However, when the blood arrives at the tissues, oxygen affinity for haemoglobin remains low, so it is easy for the oxygen to be released into the tissues. This happens when acidosis is present and there is a shift of the curve to the right.

It can be seen from the shape of the oxygen dissociation curve (Fig. 2.1) that initially there is a slight drop in saturation when there is a reduced PO_2. At a certain point (approximately 8 kPa), however, there is a sudden drop in saturation, as indicated by the steep decline in the curve. Therefore, oxygen saturation normally only drops sharply if the PO_2 is at a very low level.

A saturation of 8 kPa is the point at which the patient is in respiratory failure and is very hypoxaemic. This means that a patient's oxygen saturation may be normal or only slightly low for some time, even though their PO_2 is decreasing fairly rapidly. Therefore it is important in patients with a compromised respiratory system to carry out blood gas analysis *in conjunction* with pulse oximetry, because a decreasing PO_2 will indicate deterioration sooner than pulse oximetry alone (Jevon and Ewens, 2002).

> ### Remember
> The oxygen dissociation curve can shift
> to left or to the right (see Fig. 2.1 and Table 2.1)

Table 2.1 Shifts of the oxygen dissociation curve

	Right shift	**Left shift**
Features	Decreased oxygen–haemoglobin affinity	Increased oxygen–haemoglobin affinity
	Less oxygen carried from the lungs	More oxygen carried from the lungs
	Oxygen given up more easily in the tissues	Oxygen given up less easily in the tissues (thus tissue hypoxia may occur with normal oxygen saturation)
Causes	Acidosis Increased temperature Hypercarbia	Alkalosis Hypothermia Hypocarbia

Transport of carbon dioxide

Carbon dioxide is transported as follows:

- 7% dissolved in the plasma
- 23% carried by the globin portion of haemoglobin (this is known as carbaminohaemoglobin)
- 70% (the majority) transported as bicarbonate ions (in the plasma) back to the lungs.

Bicarbonate is formed as a result of a series of chemical reactions. First, cellular metabolism produces carbon dioxide and water. In the presence of an enzyme called carbonic anhydrase, this carbon dioxide and water combine to form carbonic acid (HCO_3). Carbonic acid is a weak acid so, to prevent acidosis, a hydrogen ion splits from the carbonic acid and is buffered by haemoglobin, and this leaves bicarbonate ions (Martini, 2006). This is shown in the equation below:

$$CO_2 + H_2O \xrightarrow{\text{Carbonic anhydrase}} H_2CO_3 \longrightarrow H + HCO_3$$

Carbon dioxide   Water   Carbonic acid   Hydrogen   Bicarbonate

Once formed, the bicarbonate ions move out of the red blood cell and into the plasma. In order to maintain electrical equilibrium, a chloride (Cl) ion moves into the cell. This is known as the chloride shift and it is illustrated in Fig. 2.2.

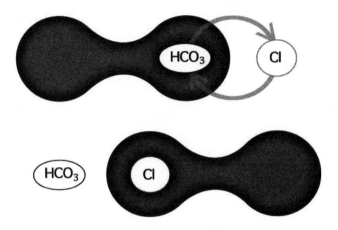

Fig. 2.2 *The chloride shift in the red blood cell.*

On reaching the lungs, the whole process is reversed so that carbon dioxide and water can be excreted. Thus it can be seen that carbon dioxide has a very important role in acid–base balance.

Consolidation

See page 73 for answers

2.1 In which two ways is oxygen transported in the blood?

2.2 What percentage of oxygen is dissolved in the plasma?

2.3 Does the oxygen carried by the haemoglobin exert a partial pressure?

2.4 What percentage of oxygen is carried by the haemoglobin?

2.5 Which of these statements is correct? (a) When PO_2 is low, oxygen is strongly affiliated with haemoglobin, or (b) when PO_2 is high, oxygen is strongly affiliated with haemoglobin.

2.6 If oxygen affiliation to haemoglobin is high, what effect will this have on oxygen delivery to the tissues?

2.7 If oxygen affiliation to haemoglobin is low, what effect does this have on oxygen delivery to the tissues?

_____

_____

2.8 If PO_2 and SaO_2 are high, does this indicate a left or right shift of the oxygen dissociation curve?

_____

2.9 If PO_2 and SaO_2 are low, does this indicate a left or right shift of the oxygen dissociation curve?

_____

2.10 What are the major causes of a right shift of the oxygen dissociation curve?

_____

_____

2.11 What are the major causes of a left shift of the oxygen dissociation curve?

_____

_____

2.12 What percentage of CO_2 is transported to the lungs in the form of bicarbonate ions?

_____

2.13 What percentage of CO_2 is dissolved in the plasma?

_____

2.14 What percentage of CO_2 is carried by haemoglobin?

_____

2.15 Which portion of the haemoglobin molecule carries CO_2?

_____

2.16 What is the name given to haemoglobin whilst carrying CO_2?

_____

2.17 When CO_2 and water combine, what is the name of the compound that is formed?

_____

2.18 Which enzyme has to be present for the formation of carbonic acid?

_____

2.19 To prevent acidosis, carbonic acid (H_2CO_3) splits into bicarbonate (HCO_3) and hydrogen (H) ions. The HCO_3 ions move out of the red blood cells into the plasma and for each one a chloride (Cl) ion moves into the cell. What is this process called?

_____

2.20 What happens to the free hydrogen ion during this process?

_____

_____

Notes

Chapter 3

Acid–base balance

To understand acid–base balance properly we need to understand where hydrogen ions come from. Before this, we need to know what acids and bases are.

What are acids and bases?

An *acid* is a substance which will *give up* hydrogen ions (pH of < 7.0) and a *base* is a substance which will *accept* hydrogen ions (pH of > 7.0). The body is very sensitive to small changes in the concentration of hydrogen ions. Any changes lead to modification of cellular function and disruption of homeostasis, and ultimately to death. Therefore, it is vital for normal cellular metabolism that the pH of the blood remains within the normal range (Martini, 2006).

Cellular metabolism produces hydrogen ions from glucose, fatty acids and amino acids. The balance of acids and bases is maintained by controlling the hydrogen ion concentration. If hydrogen ion concentration is not controlled by the body, acidosis or alkalosis will develop quickly (Bruck *et al.*, 2005).

> **Acidosis** is a process causing *acidaemia* (pH < 7.35)
>
> **Alkalosis** is a process causing *alkalaemia* (pH > 7.45)

The normal pH of blood is 7.35–7.45 and this range is maintained while the normal hydrogen ion concentration of 36–45 nmol/L (nanomoles per litre) is maintained.

Maintaining normal acid–base balance

The body has different ways of maintaining a normal acid–base balance. Briefly, these consist of:

- buffering systems
- the respiratory system, and
- the renal system.

Buffering systems

Buffers are chemical substances that act quickly to temporarily bind hydrogen ions, therefore minimising changes in the overall pH by accepting hydrogen ions when pH falls (*acidosis*) and donating hydrogen ions when pH rises (*alkalosis*). In these ways, the highly reactive excess hydrogen ions are removed from solution, but not from the body (Bruck *et al.*, 2005). There are actually three buffering systems. These are known as:

1. The carbonic acid–bicarbonate system.

2. The phosphate system.

3. The protein system (haemoglobin and plasma proteins).

A ratio of 20 to 1 (bicarbonate ions to carbonic acid ions) is required to maintain normal pH (Marieb, 2006).

Ratio for maintainence of normal pH
bicarbonate 20 : 1 carbonic acid

The buffering systems have two functions:

1. To provide an important and immediate response to potential changes in pH.

2. To prevent changes in pH until excess hydrogen ions can be excreted or bicarbonate levels restored (Gonce-Morton *et al.*, 2005).

If there are excessive changes in base or acid levels – so that the 20 to 1 ratio cannot be maintained – then a change in pH will occur.

The respiratory system

Carbon dioxide and water are produced by cellular metabolism and when carbon dioxide is dissolved in water, carbonic acid is formed. It is important that carbonic acid, having been transported back to the lungs, is excreted as carbon dioxide.

If the rate and depth of breathing are increased, more carbon dioxide will be exhaled. Therefore, excess acid (in the form of carbon dioxide) will be exhaled. This reduces the levels of carbonic acid within the body by clearing excess carbon dioxide and is effective within minutes (Marieb, 2006).

Thus the respiratory system is important in the control of acid–base balance. Furthermore, because it is able to respond quickly, it contributes to the short-term control of pH (Gonce-Morton *et al.*, 2005).

The renal system

The renal system assists in the long-term control of acid–base balance by regulating the secretion of bicarbonate ions and excreting acids. The cells of the renal tubule can alter blood pH in three ways:

1. They *secrete hydrogen ions* into the filtrate. This clears the blood of acids by making the urine more acidic.

2. They *reabsorb bicarbonate* ions.

3. They *produce new bicarbonate ions* to augment the buffering of hydrogen ions in the blood.

Consolidation

See page 74 for answers

3.1 How are hydrogen ions produced in the body?

_____

3.2 What is the definition of an acid?

_____

3.3 What is the definition of a base?

_____

3.4 What is the effect of a significant increase in hydrogen ions in the body?

_____

3.5 What is the definition of acidosis?

_____

3.6 What is the definition of alkalosis?

_____

3.7 What is the normal range of hydrogen ion concentration?

_____

3.8 In which three ways does the body maintain normal acid–base balance?

_____

_____

_____

3.9 How do buffers work?

_____

3.10 Name the buffering systems:

_____

_____

_____

3.11 What ratio of bicarbonate to carbonic acid ions is required to maintain normal blood pH?

_____

3.12 What happens if this ratio is not maintained?

_____

3.13 In what way does the respiratory system help to maintain normal acid–base balance?

_____

_____

3.14 Does the respiratory system provide short-term or long-term control of acid–base balance?

_____

3.15 In which three ways does the renal system help to maintain normal acid–base balance?

_____

_____

_____

3.16 Does the renal system provide short-term or long-term control of acid–base balance?

_____

Notes

Notes

Chapter 4

How to analyse blood gases

Now that we have looked at all the essential information we can get down to the task in hand – that is, how to analyse arterial blood gases.

Acidosis and alkalosis

Firstly, review the following pH values and decide if acidosis or alkalosis is present (*see page 75 for the answers*):

4.1 Is a pH of 7.25 acidotic or alkalotic? _____

4.2 Is a pH of 7.53 acidotic or alkalotic? _____

4.3 Is a pH of 7.48 acidotic or alkalotic? _____

4.4 Is a pH of 7.19 acidotic or alkalotic? _____

There are two types of acid–base imbalances – these are *acidosis* and *alkalosis*. Each imbalance can affect either the *respiratory* component (PCO_2) or the *metabolic* component (HCO_3). This means there can be a:

- respiratory acidosis or respiratory alkalosis, *or a*
- metabolic acidosis or metabolic alkalosis.

(Jevon and Ewens, 2002.)

Occasionally there can be a mixed imbalance, for example a respiratory acidosis with a metabolic acidosis, or a respiratory alkalosis with a metabolic alkalosis which is very dangerous for the patient. Mixed imbalances are covered in more detail later in this chapter.

A systematic approach to analysis

Here is a four-step approach to analysis.

STEP 1

Examine the PO$_2$ and SaO$_2$
Are they normal, increased or decreased?
What action needs to be taken? Is the patient receiving oxygen therapy? Are there other factors which will affect ventilation?

$\downarrow$

STEP 2

Examine the pH
Is the pH normal? Or is it high (alkalosis) or low (acidosis)?

$\downarrow$

STEP 3

Examine the PCO$_2$
Is the PCO$_2$ normal? Or is it high (respiratory acidosis) or low (respiratory alkalosis)?

$\downarrow$

STEP 4

Examine the HCO$_3$ and base excess (BE)
Are they normal? Or are they high (metabolic alkalosis) or low (metabolic acidosis)?

Considering the PCO_2 and HCO_3/BE will help you to decide if an acidosis or alkalosis is caused by a problem with the respiratory or metabolic component. Also think about what could be causing the problem and, therefore, what you could do about it.

Table 4.1 gives a brief overview of acid–base disturbances and causative factors that may be of help in your interpretation.

Table 4.1 Interpretation of blood gas results for carbon dioxide and bicarbonate

Parameter		Condition	Causative factor
PCO_2	Increased	Respiratory acidosis	Decreased elimination of CO_2
	Decreased	Respiratory alkalosis	Increased elimination of CO_2
HCO_3/BE	Increased	Metabolic alkalosis	Non-volatile acid is lost or HCO_3 is gained
	Decreased	Metabolic acidosis	Non-volatile acid is added and/or HCO_3 is used up or lost

Now you should be able to analyse the five sets of blood gases that appear on the following pages (*answers are given on pages 75–76*).

4.5 Consider these results:

pH 7.14
PO$_2$ 6.8 kPa (51 mmHg)
PCO$_2$ 7.5 kPa (56.25 mmHg)
HCO$_3$ 24 mmol/L
BE +1
SaO$_2$ 87%

What is the problem with the gases? What is a possible cause? What intervention is required?

_____

_____

_____

4.6 Consider these results:

pH 6.9
PO$_2$ 10.6 kPa (80 mmHg)
PCO$_2$ 4.5 kPa (33.75 mmHg)
HCO$_3$ 10.3 mmol/L
BE ☒7
SaO$_2$ 96%

What is the problem with the gases? What is a possible cause? What intervention is required?

_____

_____

_____

_____

4.7 Consider these results:

pH 7.51
PO$_2$ 13.6 kPa (102 mmHg)
PCO$_2$ 2.4 kPa (18 mmHg)
HCO$_3$ 24 mmol/L
BE +1
SaO$_2$ 100%

What is the problem with the gases? What is a possible cause? What intervention is required?

_____

_____

_____

4.8 Consider these results:

pH 7.52
PO$_2$ 11.0 kPa (82.5 mmHg)
PCO$_2$ 4.8 kPa (36 mmHg)
HCO$_3$ 35 mmol/L
BE +10
SaO$_2$ 96%

What is the problem with the gases? What is a possible cause? What intervention is required?

_____

_____

_____

_____

4.9 Consider these results:

pH 7.37
PO₂ 11.7 kPa (87.75 mmHg)
PCO₂ 4.8 kPa (36 mmHg)
HCO₃ 24 mmol/L
BE +1
SaO₂ 97%

What is the problem with the gases? What is a possible cause? What intervention is required?

_____

_____

_____

Compensation

Unfortunately, blood gas analysis is not always as straightforward; this is because if the pH is too high or too low, then cellular function ceases. The body therefore has natural mechanisms for keeping pH within normal limits. It is therefore possible to have widely abnormal blood gases with a relatively normal pH:

• If there is a *respiratory* acidosis (increased PCO_2) the metabolic component (bicarbonate) will increase, so increasing alkalinity to compensate and bring the pH back towards normal.
• If there is a *metabolic* acidosis (decreased bicarbonate) the respiratory component (CO_2) will decrease (by hyperventilation – to blow off CO_2 and therefore acid) to compensate and bring the pH back towards normal, and so on.

If there is sufficient compensation to bring the pH back to within normal limits, this is referred to as *full compensation*. If there is some compensation but it is insufficient to alter pH, it is known as *partial compensation*.

Bearing this in mind, you should now be able to analyse patients' results and explain what the problem is, whether there is full, partial or no compensation, what might be wrong with the patient and what intervention is required to improve his or her gases. The flowcharts in Figs 4.1 and 4.2 outline the steps of blood gas analysis. and might be of some help in your interpretation of the exercises that follow.

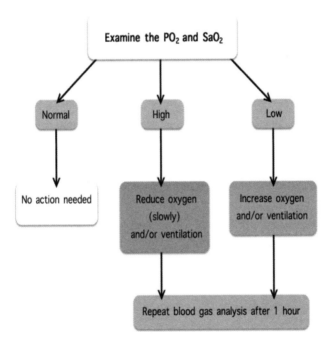

Fig. 4.1 *Interpretation of PO$_2$ and SaO$_2$.*

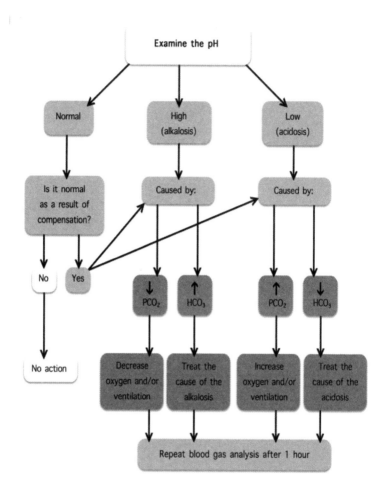

In all cases, it is important that *the cause* of the acid–base disturbance is treated rather than the disturbance itself.

Fig. 4.2 *Interpretation of acid–base status.*

To help you to determine whether the *respiratory* or *metabolic* component is causing the primary problem, consider which one (PCO_2 or HCO_3) – matches what the pH is telling you.

• Thus, if the PCO_2 is *high* (respiratory acidosis), then is the pH tending towards acidosis? If it is, there's your match – so it will be a respiratory acidosis with metabolic compensation.

• Conversely, if the HCO_3 is low (metabolic acidosis) and the pH is tending towards acidosis, that will be the primary problem and the body will ensure the other component (PCO_2) compensates (the patient will be hyperventilating in an attempt to blow off excess acid in the form of CO_2).

The information given in Table 4.2 on the next page summarises all the compensatory mechanisms that exist in response to specific disturbances. Using this informatiion, analyse the ten sets of blood gases below (*answers are given on pages 76–78*).

4.10 Consider these results:

pH 7.35
PO$_2$ 6.8 kPa (51 mmHg)
PCO$_2$ 7.5 kPa (56.25 mmHg)
HCO$_3$ 32 mmol/L
BE +6
SaO$_2$ 87%

What is the problem with the gases? Is there full, partial or no compensation? What might be wrong with the patient? What intervention is required?

_____

_____

_____

_____

Table 4.1 Overview of acid–base problems

	Causes and examples	**Compensation**
RESPIRATORY ACIDOSIS	Any condition leading to inadequate ventilation and retention of carbon dioxide, such as: • COPD (chronic obstructive pulmonary disease) • Pulmonary oedema • Under-ventilation • Over-sedation	Bicarbonate is reabsorbed by the kidneys to augment the buffering of free hydrogen ions in the blood
RESPIRATORY ALKALOSIS	Any condition leading to hyperventilation causing the excretion of too much carbon dioxide, such as: • Hysterical hyperventilation • Over (mechanical) ventilation	Re-breathing of carbon dioxide using a bag, or reduction of mechanical ventilation (by reducing volume)
METABOLIC ACIDOSIS	Any condition leading to excess acid production or loss of bicarbonate, such as: • Diabetic ketoacidosis • Renal failure • Sepsis • Cardiac arrest	Hyperventilation, in which the rate and depth of breathing are increased to blow off excess acid in the form of carbon dioxide
METABOLIC ALKALOSIS	Any condition leading to an increase in bicarbonate or loss of acids, such as: • Severe vomiting • Diuretic overdose • Antacid overdose	The rate and depth of respiration are decreased in order to retain carbon dioxide (i.e. acid)

4.11 Consider these results:

pH 7.21
PO₂ 13.6 kPa (102 mmHg)
PCO₂ 2.4 kPa (18 mmHg)
HCO₃ 14 mmol/L
BE –6
SaO₂ 100%

What is the problem with the gases? Is there full, partial or no compensation? What might be wrong with the patient? What intervention is required?

_____

_____

_____

_____

4.12 Consider these results:

pH 7.25
PO₂ 10.6 kPa (79.5 mmHg)
PCO₂ 2.3 kPa (17.25 mmHg)
HCO₃ 19.6 mmol/L
BE –3
SaO₂ 96%

What is the problem with the gases? Is there full, partial or no compensation? What might be wrong with the patient? What intervention is required?

_____

_____

_____

_____

4.13 Consider these results:

pH 7.46
PO₂ 11.0 kPa (82.5 mmHg)
PCO₂ 5.5 kPa (41.25 mmHg)
HCO₃ 29 mmol/L
BE +5
SaO₂ 96%

What is the problem with the gases? Is there full, partial or no compensation? What might be wrong with the patient? What intervention is required?

_____

_____

_____

_____

4.14 Consider these results:

pH 7.21
PO₂ 6.3 kPa (47.25 mmHg)
PCO₂ 10.0 kPa (75 mmHg)
HCO₃ 39.8 mmol/L
BE +7.7
SaO₂ 63.9%

What is the problem with the gases? Is there full, partial or no compensation? What might be wrong with the patient? What intervention is required?

_____

_____

_____

_____

4.15 Consider these results:

pH 7.28
PO₂ 8.0 kPa (60 mmHg)
PCO₂ 7.5 kPa (56.25 mmHg)
HCO₃ 24 mmol/L
BE −2
SaO₂ 94%

What is the problem with the gases? Is there full, partial or no compensation? What might be wrong with the patient? What intervention is required?

_____

_____

_____

_____

4.16 Consider these results:

pH 7.49
PO₂ 16.1 kPa (120.75 mmHg)
PCO₂ 3.1 kPa (23.25 mmHg)
HCO₃ 23 mmol/L
BE −2
SaO₂ 99%

What is the problem with the gases? Is there full, partial or no compensation? What might be wrong with the patient? What intervention is required?

_____

_____

_____

_____

4.17 Consider these results:

pH 7.29
PO₂ 11.9 kPa (89.25 mmHg)
PCO₂ 3.1 kPa (23.25 mmHg)
HCO₃ 16 mmol/L
BE −6
SaO₂ 97%

What is the problem with the gases? Is there full, partial or no compensation? What might be wrong with the patient? What intervention is required?

4.18 Consider these results:

pH 7.49
PO₂ 15.3 kPa (114.75 mmHg)
PCO₂ 1.9 kPa (14.25 mmHg)
HCO₃ 20 mmol/L
BE −6
SaO₂ 100%

What is the problem with the gases? Is there full, partial or no compensation? What might be wrong with the patient? What intervention is required?

4.19 Consider these results:

pH 7.33
PO₂ 9.2 kPa (69 mmHg)
PCO₂ 8.1 kPa (60.75 mmHg)
HCO₃ 29 mmol/L
BE +8
SaO₂ 94%

What is the problem with the gases? Is there full, partial or no compensation? What might be wrong with the patient? What intervention is required?

_____

_____

_____

_____

Over-compensation

There are occasions when there is 'over-compensation'. This over-compensation over-corrects the pH. As you become more experienced, this will become evident. Generally, you will also know the patient, or will at least have a clinical picture (that's a luxury you don't have in this workbook) and these things will guide you in determining the patient's problems.

This set of blood gases shows over-compensation
pH 7.49
PO₂ 9.2 kPa (69 mmHg)
PCO₂ 8.1 kPa (60.75 mmHg)
HCO₃ 36 mmol/L
BE +14
SaO₂ 93%

This patient has a respiratory acidosis as the PCO_2 is high and the HCO_3 has risen to such a level that the pH is demonstrating an alkalosis. The respiratory acidosis would require treatment and the metabolic acidosis would then correct itself.

Mixed imbalances

There are occasions when the patient has both a *respiratory* and a *metabolic acidosis*, or a *respiratory* and a *metabolic alkalosis*, and it is therefore impossible for the body to compensate.

> **This set of blood gases shows a patient with** *both* **a respiratory acidosis and a metabolic acidosis**
> **pH** 7.13
> **PO₂** 9.2 kPa (69 mmHg)
> **PCO₂** 8.1 kPa (60.75 mmHg)
> **HCO₃** 10 mmol/L
> **BE** −6
> **SaO₂** 93%

This patient may be suffering from an acute exacerbation of chronic bronchitis and also diabetic ketoacidosis. Physiological compensation is therefore impossible.

Medical intervention is required to overcome the rising PCO_2 and falling HCO_3. The patient would require some form of assisted ventilation and insulin therapy as well as other supportive measures.

In the following exercises you will collect and analyse six consecutive samples from a single patient, then collect and analyse samples from six different patients. You will do the same as you did with previous samples, but now you will state what action *was* taken and whether or not this worked.

Remember to discuss your findings with your mentor.

4.20 Record the results of six consecutive samples from one of your patients.

Sample 1

pH	PO$_2$	PCO$_2$	HCO$_3$	BE	SaO$_2$

Give an overview of these results:

_____

_____

_____

_____

What action was undertaken?

_____

_____

_____

What effect did the action have?

_____

_____

_____

Sample 2

pH	PO$_2$	PCO$_2$	HCO$_3$	BE	SaO$_2$

Give an overview of these results:

_____

_____

_____

_____

What action was undertaken?

_____

_____

_____

What effect did the action have?

_____

_____

_____

Sample 3

pH	PO₂	PCO₂	HCO₃	BE	SaO₂

Give an overview of these results:

_____

_____

_____

_____

What action was undertaken?

_____

_____

_____

What effect did the action have?

_____

_____

_____

Sample 4

pH	PO₂	PCO₂	HCO₃	BE	SaO₂

Give an overview of these results:

_____

_____

_____

_____

What action was undertaken?

_____

_____

_____

What effect did the action have?

_____

_____

_____

Sample 5

pH	PO$_2$	PCO$_2$	HCO$_3$	BE	SaO$_2$

Give an overview of these results:

_____

_____

_____

_____

What action was undertaken?

_____

_____

_____

What effect did the action have?

_____

_____

_____

Sample 6

pH	PO₂	PCO₂	HCO₃	BE	SaO₂

Give an overview of these results:

_____

_____

_____

_____

What action was undertaken?

_____

_____

_____

What effect did the action have?

_____

_____

_____

4.21 Record samples from six different patients as before. Discuss your findings with your mentor.

Patient 1

pH	PO₂	PCO₂	HCO₃	BE	SaO₂

Give an overview of these results:

_____

_____

_____

_____

What action was undertaken?

_____

_____

_____

What effect did the action have?

_____

_____

_____

Patient 2

pH	PO$_2$	PCO$_2$	HCO$_3$	BE	SaO$_2$

Give an overview of these results:

_____

_____

_____

_____

What action was undertaken?

_____

_____

_____

What effect did the action have?

_____

_____

_____

Patient 3

pH	PO$_2$	PCO$_2$	HCO$_3$	BE	SaO$_2$

Give an overview of these results:

_____

_____

_____

_____

What action was undertaken?

_____

_____

_____

What effect did the action have?

_____

_____

_____

Patient 4

pH	PO$_2$	PCO$_2$	HCO$_3$	BE	SaO$_2$

Give an overview of these results:

_____

_____

_____

_____

What action was undertaken?

_____

_____

_____

What effect did the action have?

_____

_____

_____

Patient 5

pH	PO$_2$	PCO$_2$	HCO$_3$	BE	SaO$_2$

Give an overview of these results:

_____

_____

_____

_____

What action was undertaken?

_____

_____

_____

What effect did the action have?

_____

_____

_____

Patient 6

pH	PO$_2$	PCO$_2$	HCO$_3$	BE	SaO$_2$

Give an overview of these results:

_____

_____

_____

_____

What action was undertaken?

_____

_____

_____

What effect did the action have?

_____

_____

_____

4.22 Fill in the table below, using arrows to show how each parameter is affected in each condition – using arrows to show increases and decreases and the letter N for normal values. (*Answers are given on page 79.*)

Condition	pH	PCO$_2$	HCO$_3$	BE
Respiratory acidosis with no compensation				
Respiratory alkalosis with no compensation				
Metabolic acidosis with no compensation				
Metabolic alkalosis with no compensation				
Respiratory acidosis with partial compensation				
Respiratory alkalosis with partial compensation				
Metabolic acidosis with partial compensation				
Metabolic alkalosis with partial compensation				
Respiratory acidosis with full compensation				
Respiratory alkalosis with full compensation				
Metabolic acidosis with full compensation				
Metabolic alkalosis with full compensation				

N.B. A severe metabolic alkalosis is not usually fully compensated by the body because this would mean significantly slowing respiration to increase the PCO$_2$ – the body knows this is not a good idea!

Notes

Chapter 5

How to obtain an arterial sample of blood

There are two methods of sampling. Samples can be taken by arterial puncture (otherwise known as a 'stab') or from an indwelling arterial line.

Sampling methods

Only health professionals who have had specific training should undertake an arterial puncture. If you are able to do this in your clinical area, you will be given appropriate training and undertake an assessment before carrying out the procedure. Make sure you follow local procedure whenever carrying out an arterial puncture.

Samples are usually taken from the radial artery because it is easily accessible, although the brachial and femoral arteries are sometimes used. Use of the femoral artery poses a potential increase in infection risk because of its position. If you use the radial artery, then you should (before performing an arterial puncture or inserting an indwelling arterial line) carry out an Allen's test to make sure the collateral circulation to the hand is adequate for maintaining perfusion (Haworth *et al.*, 2004). See Fig. 5.1.

Carrying out the Allen's test

Occlude the radial and ulnar arteries until the hand blanches (usually 10 to 30 seconds), then release the pressure on the ulnar artery. Colour should return to the hand within 15 seconds.

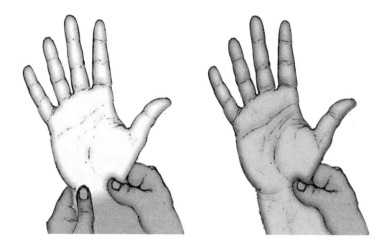

Fig. 5.1 *Allen's test. Occlude the radial and ulnar arteries (left). Pallor is produced as a result of occlusion. When the ulnar artery is released, colour should return to normal within seconds (right). If not, use another site.*

If colour does not return to the hand within 15 seconds, an alternative site should be used for the arterial puncture or for inserting the arterial line.

Once the sample has been obtained, apply pressure to the puncture site for 3–5 minutes to avoid bleeding (Haworth *et al.*, 2004). If the patient is receiving anticoagulant therapy or has a coagulopathy (clotting disorder), it may be necessary to apply pressure for longer. Whenever possible, a sample should be taken from an indwelling arterial line, although it is not necessary to insert such a line for a one-off sample.

Taking blood from an indwelling arterial line

You will need the following equipment:

- a 5-mL syringe
- a heparinised syringe
- alcohol swabs
- a sterile cap.

The following procedure is based on guidelines by Driscoll *et al.* (1997).

1. Collect the necessary equipment and wash your hands to ensure all equipment is available and maintain a clean environment.

2. Inform the patient of your actions to obtain consent and cooperation.

3. Ensure the three-way tap is closed to air. This prevents backflow of blood.

4. Remove the cap from the three-way tap, wipe the port with an alcohol swab and connect a 5-mL syringe to gain access to the artery and maintain sterility.

5. Turn the three-way tap to gain access to the artery and withdraw sufficient waste to ensure the sample is purely blood with no diluent (usually approximately 5 mL). This ensures that the blood sent for analysis does not contain any flush solution from the arterial line.

6. Turn the three-way tap so that it is off to the syringe and disconnect the syringe, ensuring safe disposal.

7. Connect the heparinised syringe and turn the three-way tap to gain access to the artery and the arterial blood.

8. Aspirate approximately 2 mL of blood. Do this slowly to prevent arterial spasm (Mallett and Dougherty, 2000).

9. Turn the three-way tap so it is off to the artery. This prevents blood loss.

10. Disconnect the syringe and apply the sterile cap to the port (to maintain sterility).

11. Flush the tubing until the fluid runs clear, to maintain patency of the line.

> **N.B.** This procedure is for guidance *only*. You should always follow local policy and procedure. Carry out blood gas analysis according to the instructions provided by the supplier of the equipment.

Once the results are available, ensure they are appropriately documented and inform medical staff if necessary.

Consolidation

See page 80 for the answers

5.1 In which two ways may a sample of arterial blood be obtained?

_____

_____

5.2 Which arteries may be used for obtaining blood samples?

_____

5.3 Why is the femoral artery avoided if possible?

_____

5.4 Why is the radial artery the preferred site for arterial puncture?

_____

5.5 Which test should be carried out prior to performing a puncture of the radial artery?

_____

5.6 Why does this test need to be carried out?

_____

5.7 How is this test carried out?

_____

5.8 For how long should pressure be applied to the puncture site following an arterial puncture?

_____

5.9 What equipment is needed to obtain a blood sample from an arterial line?

_____

5.10 Approximately how many millilitres of blood should be withdrawn via the arterial line prior to obtaining the blood sample for analysis?

_____

5.11 Why does this need to be done?

_____

_____

5.12 Why does the sample of arterial blood need to be aspirated slowly?

_____

_____

5.13 Once you have obtained the results of the blood gases, what two actions must be undertaken?

_____

_____

_____

5.14 Under the supervision of your mentor, take five samples of blood from an arterial line, following local procedure. Record your progress in the table below. Discuss any issues with your mentor.

	Date	**Comments**	**Signature of mentor**
Sample 1			
Sample 2			
Sample 3			
Sample 4			
Sample 5			

Notes

Notes

References

Bruck, L., Donofrio, J., Munden, J. and Thompson, G. (eds) (2005). *Anatomy and Physiology Made Incredibly Easy*, 2nd edn. London: ippincott, Williams and Wilkins..

Driscoll, P., Brown, T. and Gwinnutt, C. (1997). *A Simple Guide to Blood Gas Analysis*. London: BMJ Publishing Group.

Gonce-Morton, P., Fontaine, D. K., Hudak, C.M. and Gallo, B.M. (2005). *Critical Care Nursing: A Holistic Approach*, 8th edn. London: Lippincott, Williams and Wilkins.

Haworth, K., Mayer, B.H., Mundon, J., Munson, C., Schaeffer, L. and Wittig, P. (eds) (2004). *Critical Care Nursing Made Incredibly Easy*. London: Lippincott, Williams and Wilkins.

Janson-Cohen, B. (2005). *Memmler's The Human Body in Health and Disease*, 10th edn. London: Lippincott, Williams and Wilkins:.

Jevon, P. and Ewens, B. (eds) (2002). *Monitoring the Critically Ill Patient*. Oxford: Blackwell Science.

Mallett, J. and Dougherty, L. (eds) (2000). *The Royal Marsden Hospital Manual of Clinical Nursing Procedures*. Oxford: Blackwell Science.

Marieb, E.N. (2006). *Essentials of Human Anatomy and Physiology*, 8th edn. London: Pearson.

Martini, F.H. (2006). *Fundamentals of Anatomy and Physiology*, 7th edn. London: Pearson.

Mattson-Porth, C. (2005). *Pathophysiology: Concepts of Altered Health States*, 7th edn. London: Lippincott, Williams and Wilkins.

Resuscitation Council UK (2000). *Advanced Life Support Manual*, 7th edn. London: Resuscitation Council.

Shoulders-Odom, B. (2000). Using an algorithm to interpret arterial blood gases. Dimensions of Critical Care Nursing, **19**(1), 36.

Viney, C. (1999). *Nursing the Critically Ill*. London: Bailliere Tindall.

Answers and Teaching Notes

1: The parameters

1.1 The parameters and their normal ranges are:
pH 7.35–7.45 (no units)
PO_2 10.6–13.3 kPa (or 80–100 mmHg)
PCO_2 4.6–6.0 kPa (or 35–45 mmHg)
HCO_3 22–26 mmol/L
BE –2 to +2.
SaO_2 – normal value is 97 %.

1.2 Acidity or alkalinity of a substance.

1.3 Acidic.

1.4 Alkaline.

1.5 Water.

1.6 Slightly alkaline.

1.7 Hydrogen.

1.8 Arterial.

1.9 Alveolar.

1.10 Partial pressure.

1.11 Dalton's Law states that each gas in a mixture exerts a partial pressure relative to its concentration in the mixture. Adding together all of the partial pressures exerted by each gas gives the sum total pressure of the mixture.

1.12 74.85 mmHg.

1.13 6.04 kPa.

1.14 No.

1.15 Carbonic acid.

1.16 70 %.

1.17 High.

1.18 Low.

1.19 By haemoglobin.

1.20 Iron.

1.21 Protein.

1.22 Four.

1.23 75 %.

1.24 1.34 mL.

1.25 Patient 2.

2: Gas transport

2.1 (i) Dissolved in the plasma and (ii) attached to haemoglobin.

2.2 Less than 3%.

2.3 No.

2.4 97%.

2.5 (b).

2.6 Oxygen delivery is reduced as it is more difficult for oxygen to be released from haemoglobin.

2.7 Oxygen is released more easily from haemoglobin.

2.8 Left shift.

2.9 Right shift.

2.10 Acidosis, increased temperature and hypercarbia.

2.11 Alkalosis, hypothermia and hypocarbia.

2.12 70%.

2.13 7%.

2.14 23%.

2.15 The globin portion.

2.16 Carbaminohaemoglobin.

2.17 Carbonic acid.

2.18 Carbonic anhydrase.

2.19 Chloride shift.

2.20 It is buffered by haemoglobin.

3: Acid–base balance

3.1 By cellular metabolism from glucose, fatty acids and amino acids.

3.2 A substance that gives up hydrogen ions (pH < 7.0).

3.3 A substance that accepts hydrogen ions (pH > 7.0).

3.4 Increased hydrogen ion concentration leads to modification of cellular function and disruption of homeostasis, ultimately leading to death.

3.5 A process causing acidaemia (pH < 7.35).

3.6 A process causing alkalaemia (pH > 7.45).

3.7 36–45 nmol/L.

3.8 (i) Buffering systems; (ii) the respiratory system; (iii) the renal system.

3.9 Buffers are chemical substances that act quickly to temporarily bind hydrogen ions, therefore minimising changes in overall pH by accepting hydrogen ions when pH falls (acidosis) and donating hydrogen ions when pH rises (alkalosis).

3.10 The carbonic acid–bicarbonate buffer system, the phosphate buffer system; and protein buffer system (haemoglobin and plasma proteins).

3.11 20 to 1 (20 bicarbonate ions to 1 carbonic acid ion).

3.12 Excessive changes in base or acid (so the ratio of 20 to 1 cannot be maintained) result in a change in pH.

3.13 If the rate and depth of breathing are increased, more carbon dioxide will be exhaled, therefore excess acid (in the form of carbon dioxide) is exhaled. This reduces the levels of carbonic acid within the body and is effective within minutes.

3.14 Short term.

3.15 (i) By secreting hydrogen ions into the filtrate, which rids the blood of acids by making the urine more acidic; (ii) by reabsorbing bicarbonate ions; (iii) by producing new bicarbonate ions to augment the buffering of hydrogen ions in the blood.

3.16 Long term.

4: How to analyse blood gases

4.1 Acidotic.

4.2 Alkalotic.

4.3 Alkalotic.

4.4 Acidotic.

4.5 This is respiratory acidosis. The gases show a decrease in pH, an increase in PCO_2 and a decrease in PO_2 and therefore show respiratory acidosis with hypoxia. Also demonstrated is a left shift of the oxygen dissociation curve (PO_2 and SaO_2 are low). The gases would have been taken from a patient with respiratory failure, or possibly COPD (chronic obstructive pulmonary disease). The patient will require oxygen therapy and possibly assisted ventilation (with caution if it is a COPD patient). If the patient is already on a ventilator, the ventilation should be increased by giving a larger minute or tidal volume so that more carbon dioxide will be exhaled.

4.6 This is metabolic acidosis. The gases show a decrease in pH and a decrease in HCO_3 and BE and therefore show a metabolic acidosis. A metabolic acidosis may be caused by diabetic ketoacidosis (DKA). The intervention required would be control of DKA with insulin – all other problems will then resolve. Other causes may be renal failure or sepsis, in which case the cause needs to be treated to correct the acidosis.

4.7 This is respiratory alkalosis. The gases show an increase in pH and a decrease in PCO_2 and therefore show a respiratory alkalosis. If the patient is on a ventilator, the ventilation should be decreased by reducing the minute or tidal volume so that the PCO_2 can rise to normal (unless the patient is being purposely hyperventilated). If the patient is not ventilated, then he is probably hysterically hyperventilating and should be given a paper bag to breathe into; by re-breathing carbon dioxide, the PCO_2 will rise to normal and the patient will become calm.

4.8 This is metabolic acidosis. The gases show an increase in pH and an increase in HCO_3 and BE and therefore show a metabolic alkalosis. The major causes are hyperemesis (severe vomiting), which causes loss of acid from the body, and overdose of antacids, which adds excess base to the body. Any interventions are aimed at treating the cause of the alkalosis.

4.9 These gases are perfect!

4.10 This is hypoxia with a fully compensated respiratory acidosis. The gases show a normal pH so it would seem there is no acidosis or alkalosis present, however all other parameters are abnormal, so there is indeed a problem. The PCO_2 is raised, indicating a respiratory acidosis, and the bicarbonate is raised, indicating a metabolic alkalosis. The pH is within the normal range but it tends towards acidosis (it is lower than 7.4) so there is a match with the PCO_2 as the PCO_2 is demonstrating acidosis. So the primary problem is caused by the raised PCO_2 and the raised bicarbonate is the compensating factor, indicating that there is renal compensation. Further, the PO_2 and SaO_2 are low, indicating hypoxia and a right shift of the oxygen dissociation curve, which in turn indicates that the patient's ventilation is inadequate and hence carbon dioxide is being retained.

4.11 This is a partially compensated metabolic acidosis. The gases show a decrease in pH and therefore the patient is clearly acidotic. There is also a decrease in HCO_3 and BE, which shows a metabolic acidosis, but the PCO_2 is low, which indicates a respiratory alkalosis. The pH and HCO_3 match in what they are demonstrating – that is, acidosis. Thus, the primary problem is a metabolic acidosis and the compensatory mechanism is the reduction in PCO_2 as the patient is hyperventilating in response to the metabolic acidosis in an attempt to exhale excess acid. As the pH has not returned to within normal limits, the compensation is partial. The cause of the acidosis should be treated, rather than the acidosis itself.

4.12 This is a partially compensated metabolic acidosis. As with the gases in 4.11, these show a decrease in pH and therefore the patient is clearly acidotic. There is also a decrease in HCO_3 and BE, showing a metabolic acidosis, but the PCO_2 is low, indicating a respiratory alkalosis. The pH and HCO_3 match in what they are demonstrating – that is, acidosis. Thus, the primary problem is a metabolic acidosis and the compensatory mechanism is the reduction in PCO_2 as the patient is hyperventilating in response to the metabolic acidosis, in an attempt to exhale excess acid. As the pH has not returned to within normal limits, the compensation is partial. The cause of the acidosis should be treated, rather than the acidosis itself.

4.13 This is an uncompensated metabolic alkalosis. The gases show an increase in pH and an increase in HCO_3 and BE. Therefore a metabolic alkalosis is present. The PCO_2 is not above the upper limit of normal, so there is no compensation. The cause of the alkalosis should be treated, rather than the alkalosis itself.

4.14 This is hypoxia with a partially compensated respiratory acidosis. The gases show a low pH, demonstrating an acidosis, and all other parameters are also abnormal. The PCO_2 is raised, indicating a respiratory acidosis which matches the pH (i.e. acidosis) so the respiratory acidosis is the primary problem. The bicarbonate is raised, indicating a metabolic alkalosis, and demonstrates renal compensation, although it is only partial compensation as the pH remains low. Also the PO_2 and SaO_2 are low, indicating hypoxia, and a right shift of the oxygen dissociation curve indicates that the patient's ventilation is inadequate and hence is retaining carbon dioxide. A patient with such blood gases would be seriously ill and would require assisted ventilation.

4.15 This is hypoxia and respiratory acidosis with no compensation. These gases show a low pH, demonstrating an acidosis. The PCO_2 is raised, indicating a respiratory acidosis which matches the pH (that is, acidosis) so the respiratory acidosis is the primary problem. The bicarbonate is normal however, so there is no compensation at present. The PO_2 and SaO_2 are low, indicating hypoxia and a right shift of the oxygen dissociation curve, showing that the patient's ventilation is inadequate and hence carbon dioxide is being retained. Although not as severe those in 4.14, a patient with such blood gases would be seriously ill and would require assisted ventilation.

4.16 This is a respiratory alkalosis with no compensation. The gases show an increase in pH, so alkalosis is present. There is a decreased PCO_2 and this indicates a respiratory alkalosis. The HCO_3 is normal and therefore there is no compensation. If the patient is on a ventilator, the ventilation should be decreased by reducing the minute or tidal volume so that the PCO_2 can rise to normal (unless the patient is being deliberately hyperventilated). If the patient is not ventilated, then he is probably hysterically hyperventilating and should be given a paper bag to breathe into; by re-breathing carbon dioxide, the PCO_2 will return to normal.

4.17 This is a partially compensated metabolic acidosis. The gases show a decrease in pH and therefore the patient is acidotic. There is also a decrease in HCO_3 and BE, indicating a metabolic acidosis, but the PCO_2 is low, demonstrating a respiratory alkalosis. The pH and HCO_3 match the pH, both showing acidosis. Thus, the primary problem is a metabolic acidosis and the compensatory mechanism is the reduction in PCO_2 as the patient is hyperventilating in response to the metabolic acidosis in an attempt to exhale excess acid. As the pH has not returned to within normal limits, the compensation is partial. The cause of the acidosis should be treated, rather than the acidosis itself.

4.18 This is a partially compensated respiratory alkalosis. The gases show an increase in pH and a decrease in PCO_2 and therefore demonstrate a respiratory alkalosis. The HCO_3 is a little low so there is some compensation, although this is only partial as the pH remains high. It is likely that you would only see blood gases like this if the patient is on a ventilator and has been over-ventilated for some time. The ventilation should be decreased by reducing the minute or tidal volume so that the PCO_2 can increase.

4.19 This is a partially compensated respiratory acidosis. These gases show a low pH, demonstrating an acidosis. All other parameters are also abnormal. The PCO_2 is raised, indicating a respiratory acidosis and matches the pH (showing acidosis), so the respiratory acidosis is the primary problem. The bicarbonate is raised, indicating a metabolic alkalosis (which is the compensating factor), although it is only partial compensation as the pH remains lower than normal. Also the PO_2 and SaO_2 are low, indicating hypoxia, and a right shift of the oxygen dissociation curve indicates that the patient's ventilation is inadequate and hence carbon dioxide is being retained.

4.20 Discuss your findings with your mentor.

4.21 Discuss your findings with your mentor.

4.22 Parameters in each condition will be increased (↑) or decreased (↓) or normal (N) as shown below.

Condition	pH	PCO$_2$	HCO$_3$	BE
Respiratory acidosis with no compensation	↓	↑	N	N
Respiratory alkalosis with no compensation	↑	↓	N	N
Metabolic acidosis with no compensation	↓	N	↓	↓
Metabolic alkalosis with no compensation	↑	N	↑	↑
Respiratory acidosis with partial compensation	↓	↑	↑	↑
Respiratory alkalosis with partial compensation	↑	↓	↓	↓
Metabolic acidosis with partial compensation	↓	↓	↓	↓
Metabolic alkalosis with partial compensation	↑	↑	↑	↑
Respiratory acidosis with full compensation	N	↑	↑	↑
Respiratory alkalosis with full compensation	N	↓	↓	↓
Metabolic acidosis with full compensation	N	↓	↓	↓
Metabolic alkalosis with full compensation	N	↑	↑	↑

5: How to obtain an arterial blood sample

5.1 Via an arterial puncture (stab) or from an indwelling arterial line.

5.2 The radial, brachial and femoral (avoid this if possible).

5.3 There is an increased risk of infection because of its position.

5.4 It is the most accessible.

5.5 The Allen's test.

5.6 To ensure the collateral circulation is adequate to maintain perfusion.

5.7 Occlude the radial and ulnar arteries until the hand blanches (usually takes 10 to 30 seconds). Then release the pressure on the ulnar artery. Colour should return within 15 seconds; if it does not, choose an alternative site.

5.8 For 3 to 5 minutes, or longer if the patient has a coagulopathy or is receiving anticoagulant therapy.

5.9 Alcohol swabs, a 5-mL syringe, a heparinised syringe and a sterile cap.

5.10 5 mL.

5.11 To ensure the sample for analysis does not contain any diluent from the arterial line as this would affect the results.

5.12 To avoid arterial spasm.

5.13 You should (i) document the results and (ii) inform medical staff if necessary.

5.14 Discuss your findings with your mentor.

Index

Index